Don't have a COW! for lunch.

Every bite counts.

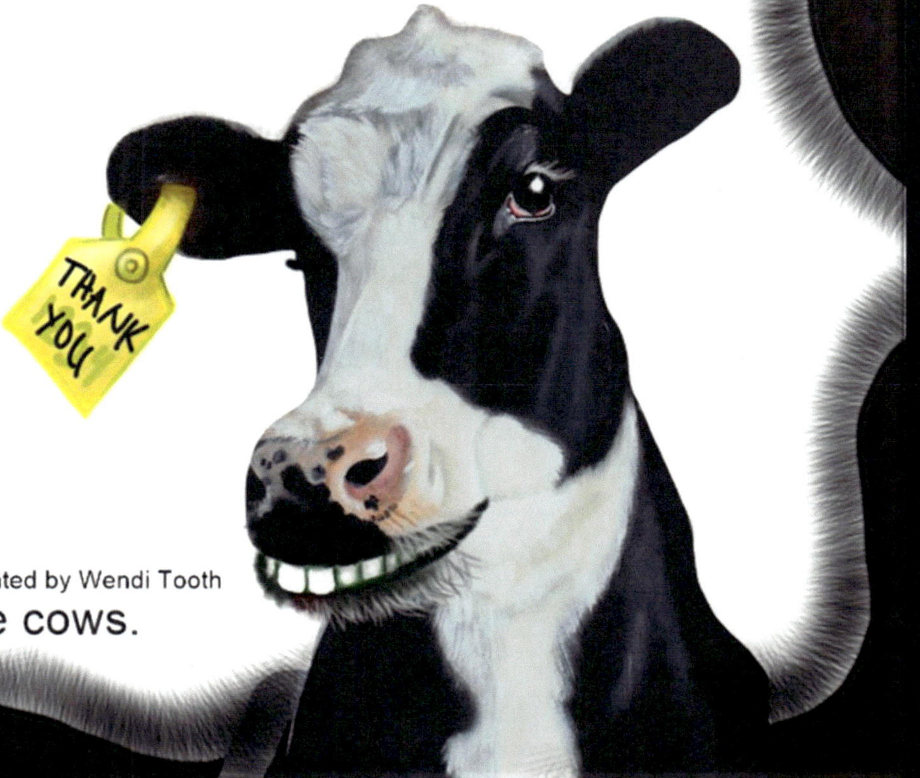

written and illustrated by Wendi Tooth

for the cows.

ISBN: 978-1-7356284-0-0

This is for the cows in factory farming,
You need to know it's not just them we are harming.

Earth is at a vital point in history,
That time to change is no longer a mystery.

So follow along and take note of every fact,
Of how dairy and meat have a
global impact.

The cows want to live just like you and me,
They bond with their calves like a newborn baby.

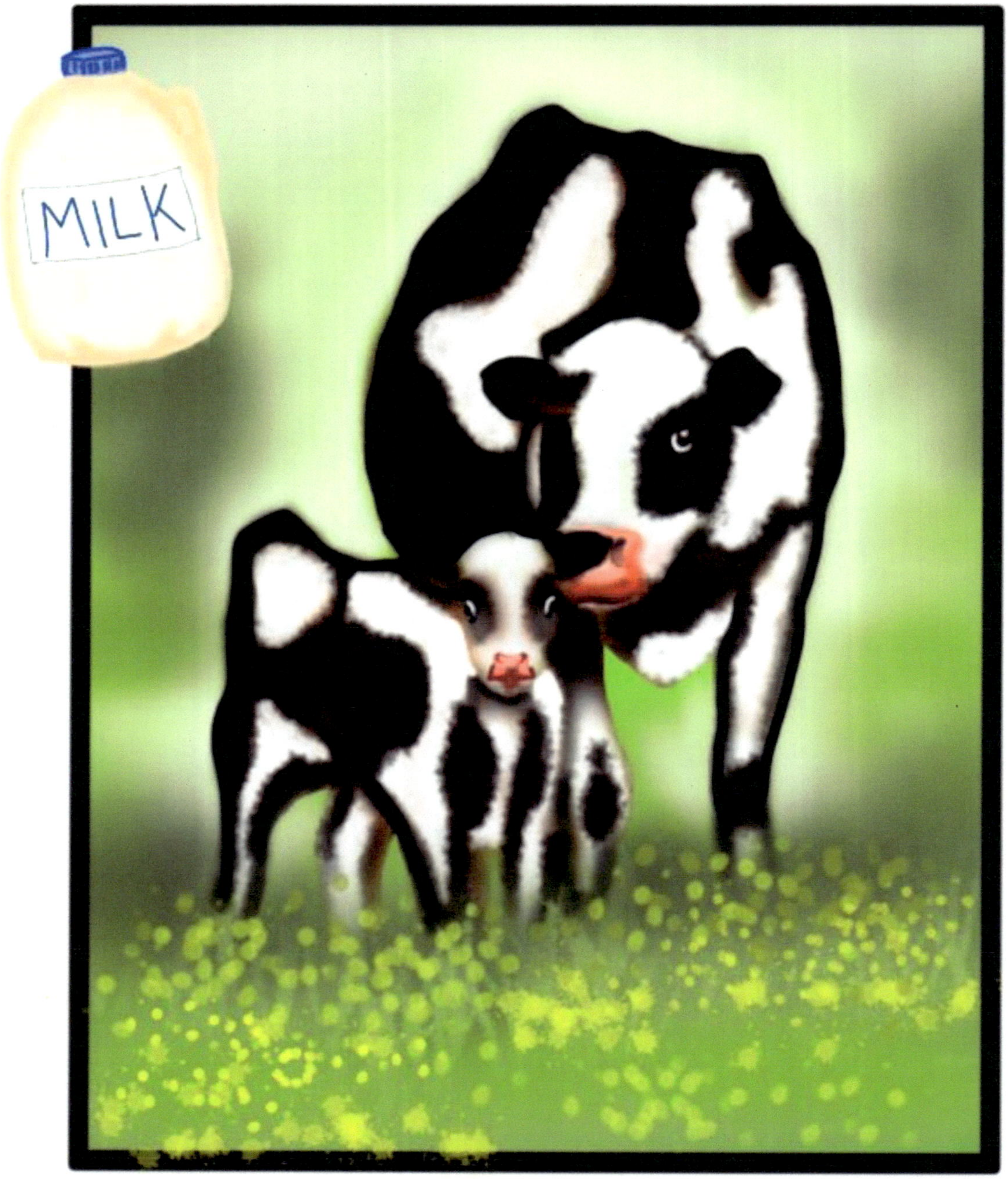

The life of the calf, alone and scary,

Taken from Mom so we can have dairy.

The farmers come and take them away,
For every dairy product, a life has to pay.

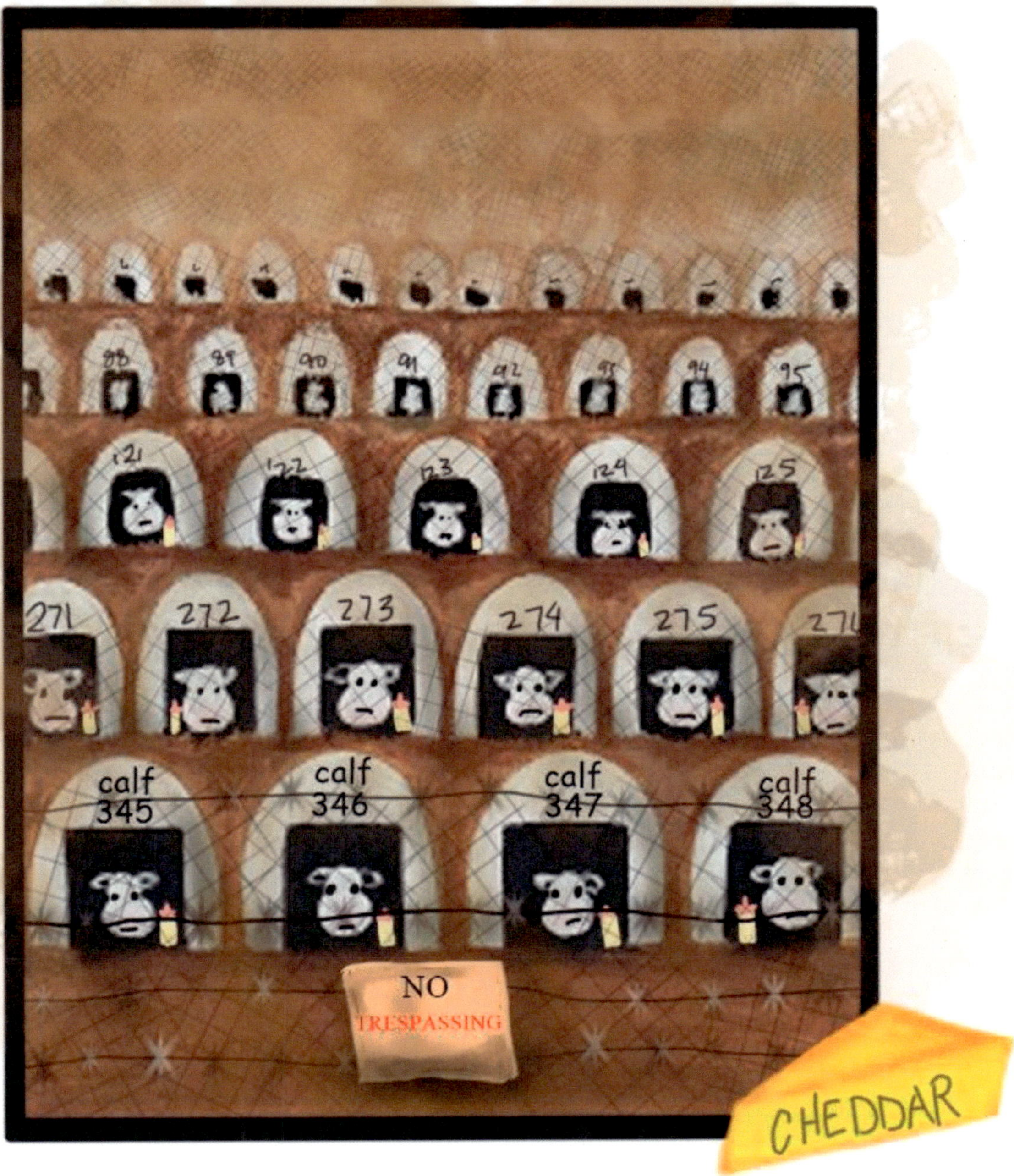

A few years later, Mom has no use,
Thrown away after a life of abuse.

They stand outside in the cold, rain, and heat,

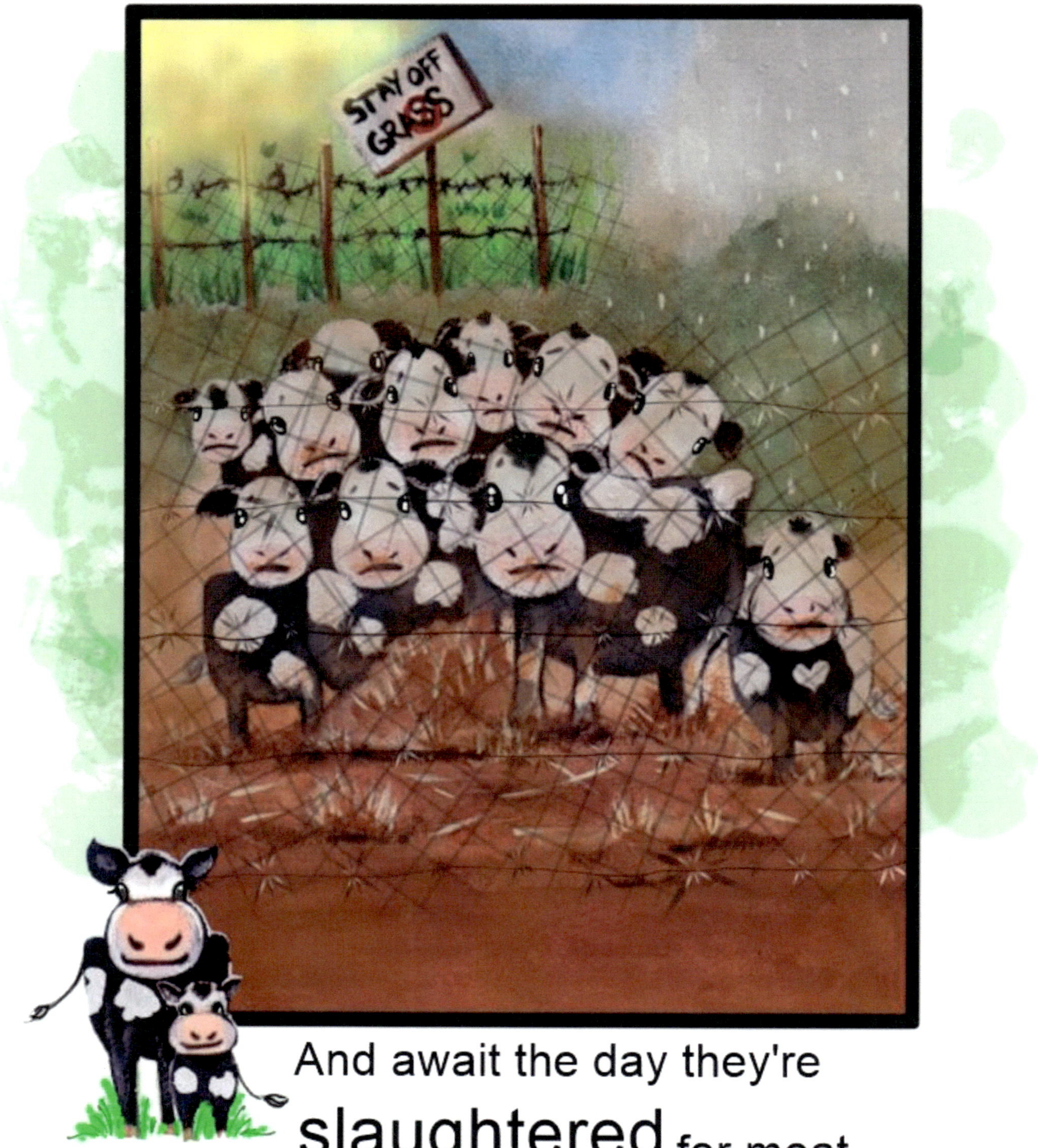

And await the day they're **slaughtered** for meat.

They keep the truth behind well scripted lies,
A life of only pain before their demise.

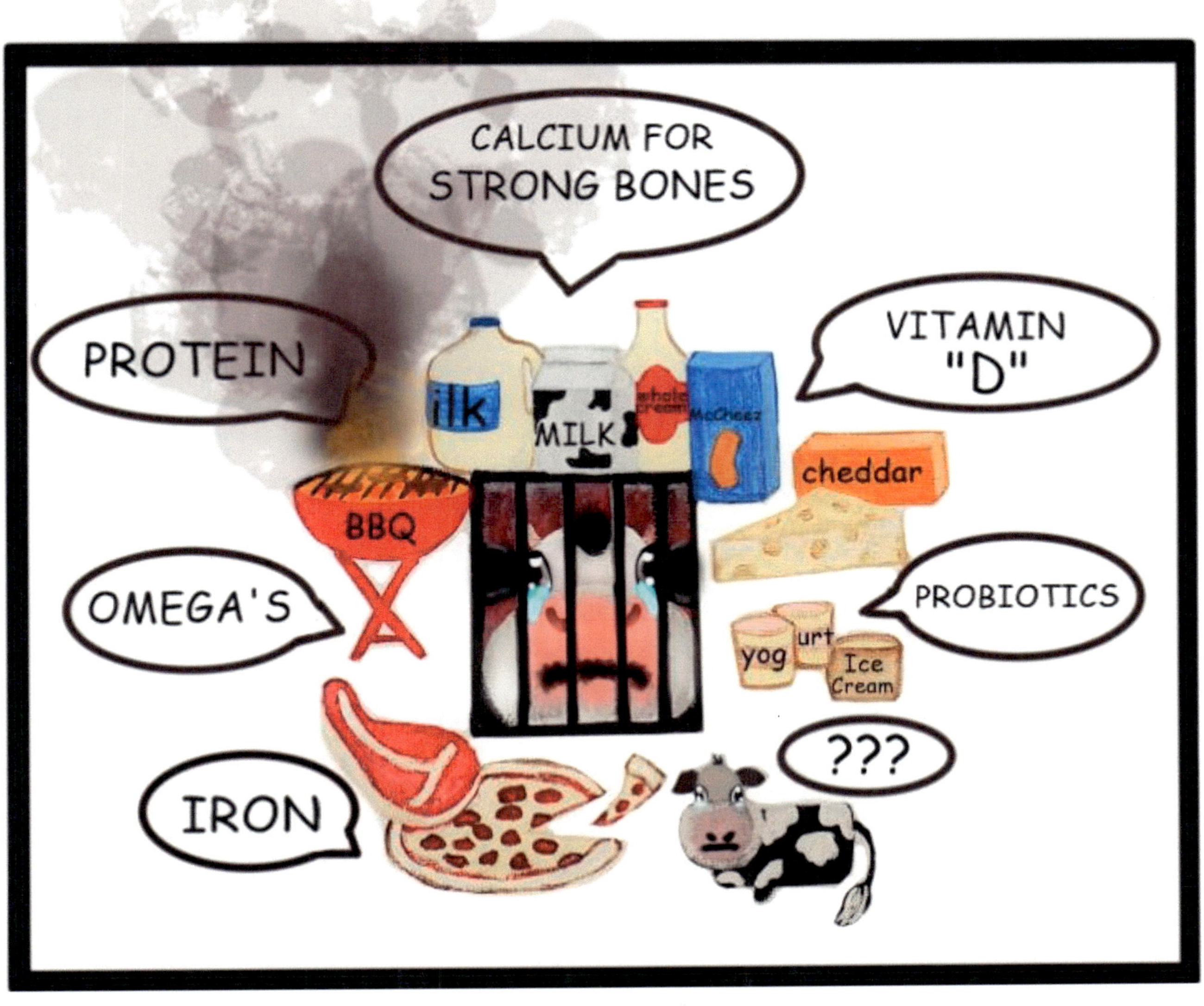

A cry for mercy before the last breath,
This is all they will know before their death.

The companies have a license to kill,
This secret hidden behind an
Ag Gag bill.

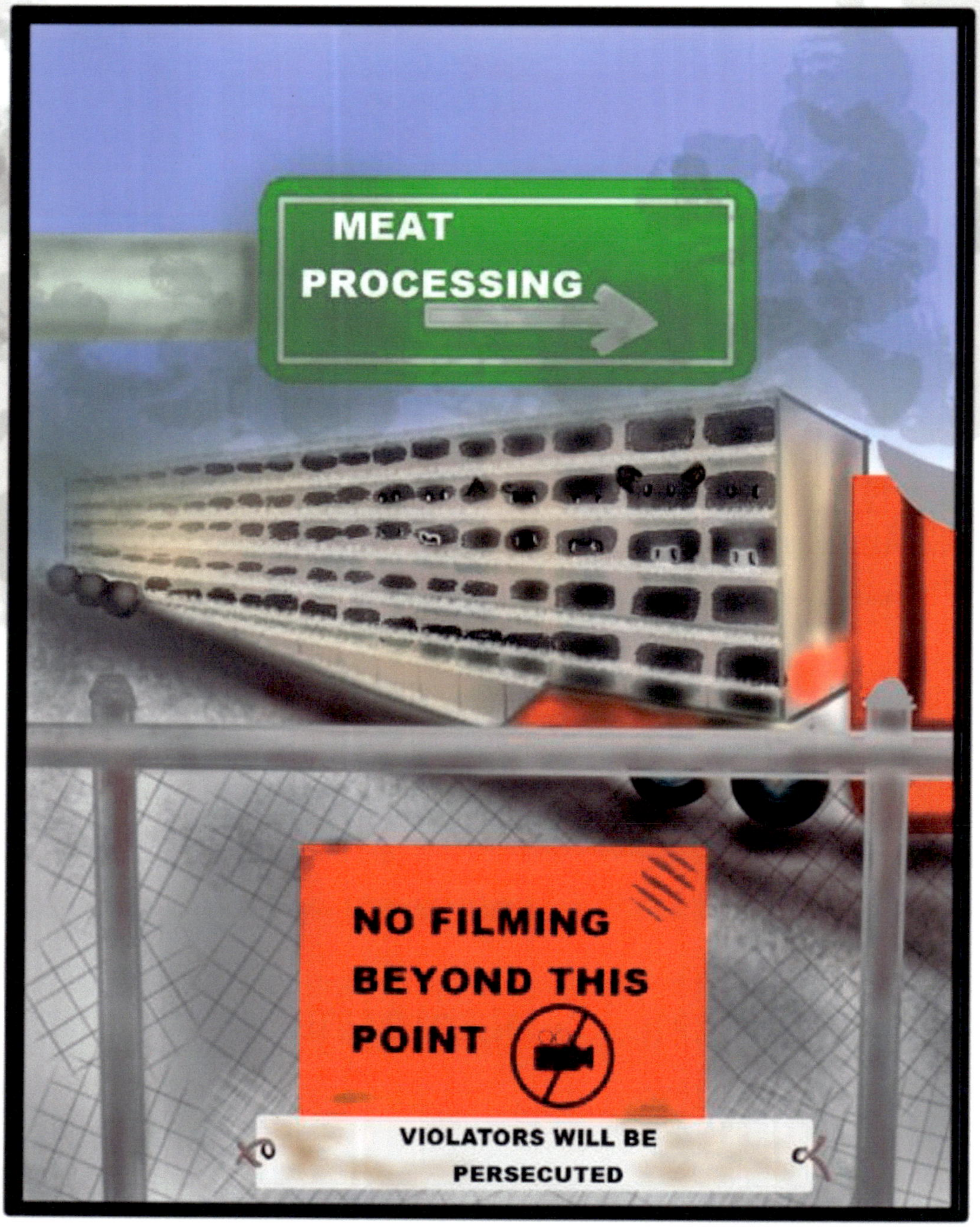

Feeding these cows takes a lot of grass,
But the process creates too much
greenhouse gas.

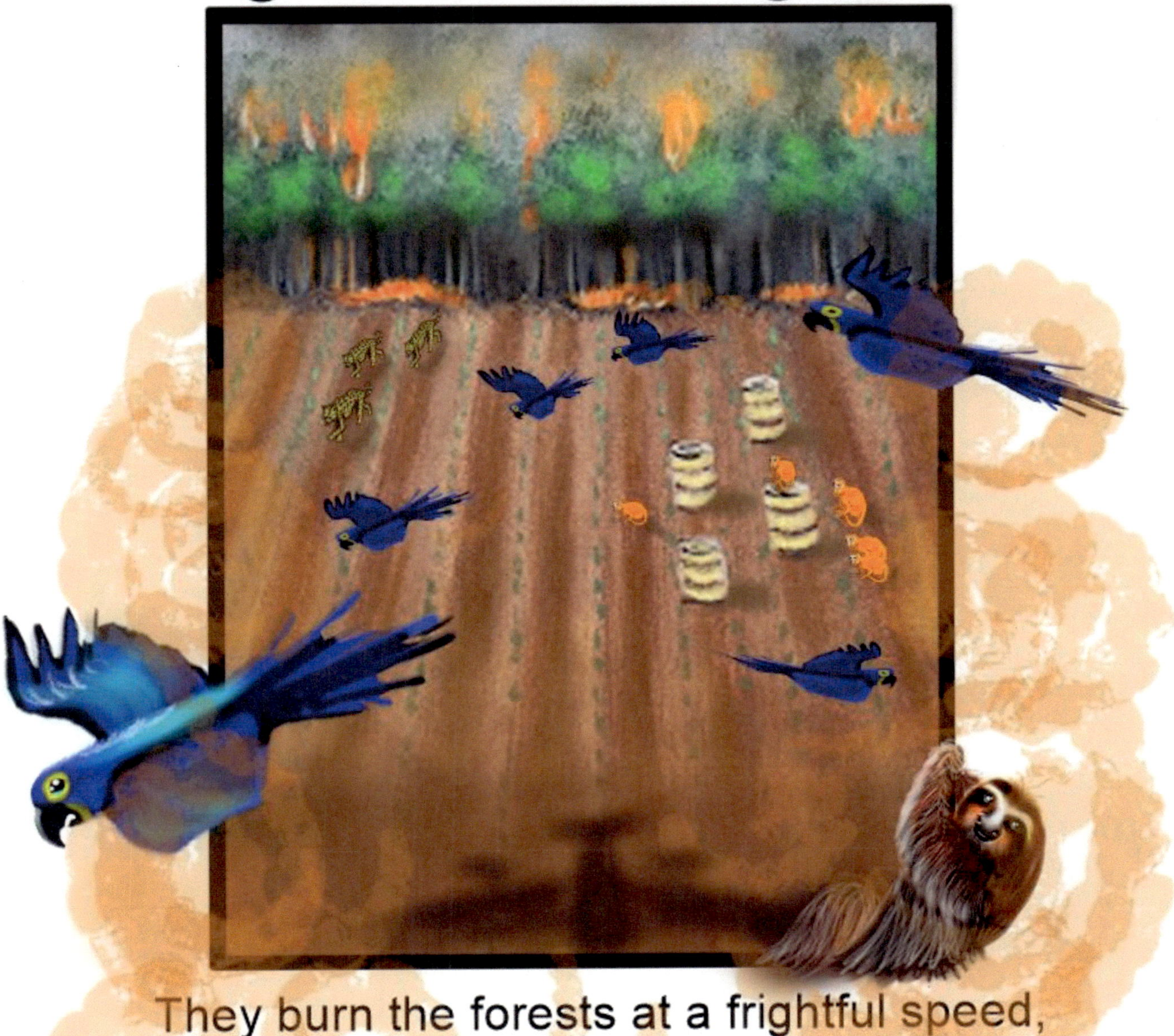

They burn the forests at a frightful speed,
causing **species extinction**
to grow the feed.

The pollution hurts all of Earth's species,
No land to spare, the sea gets the feces.

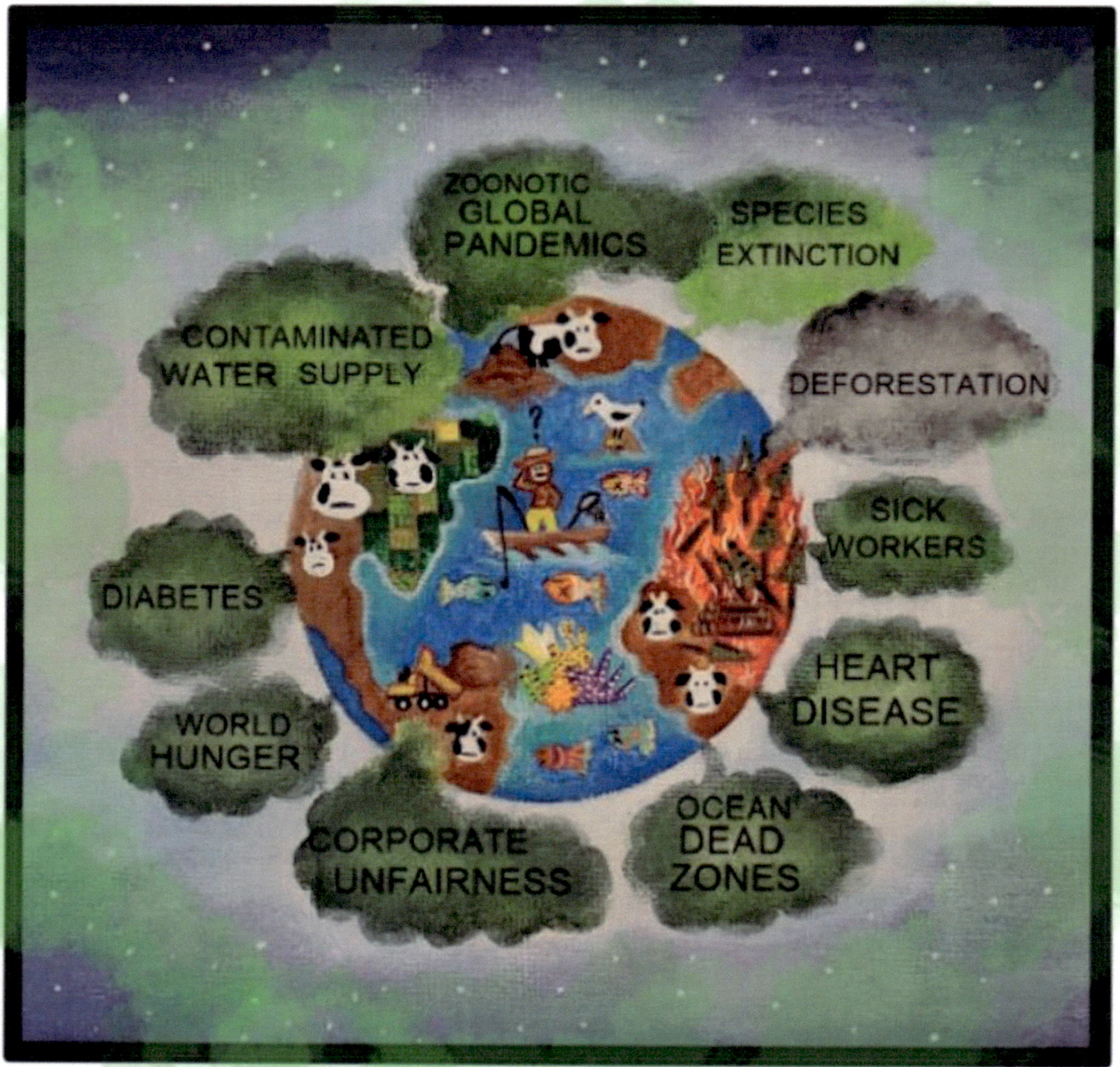

Why are they dumping poop in the ocean?
To keep the cycle always in motion.

Restaurants and schools both claim to need meat,

But at this pace, the world will

overheat!

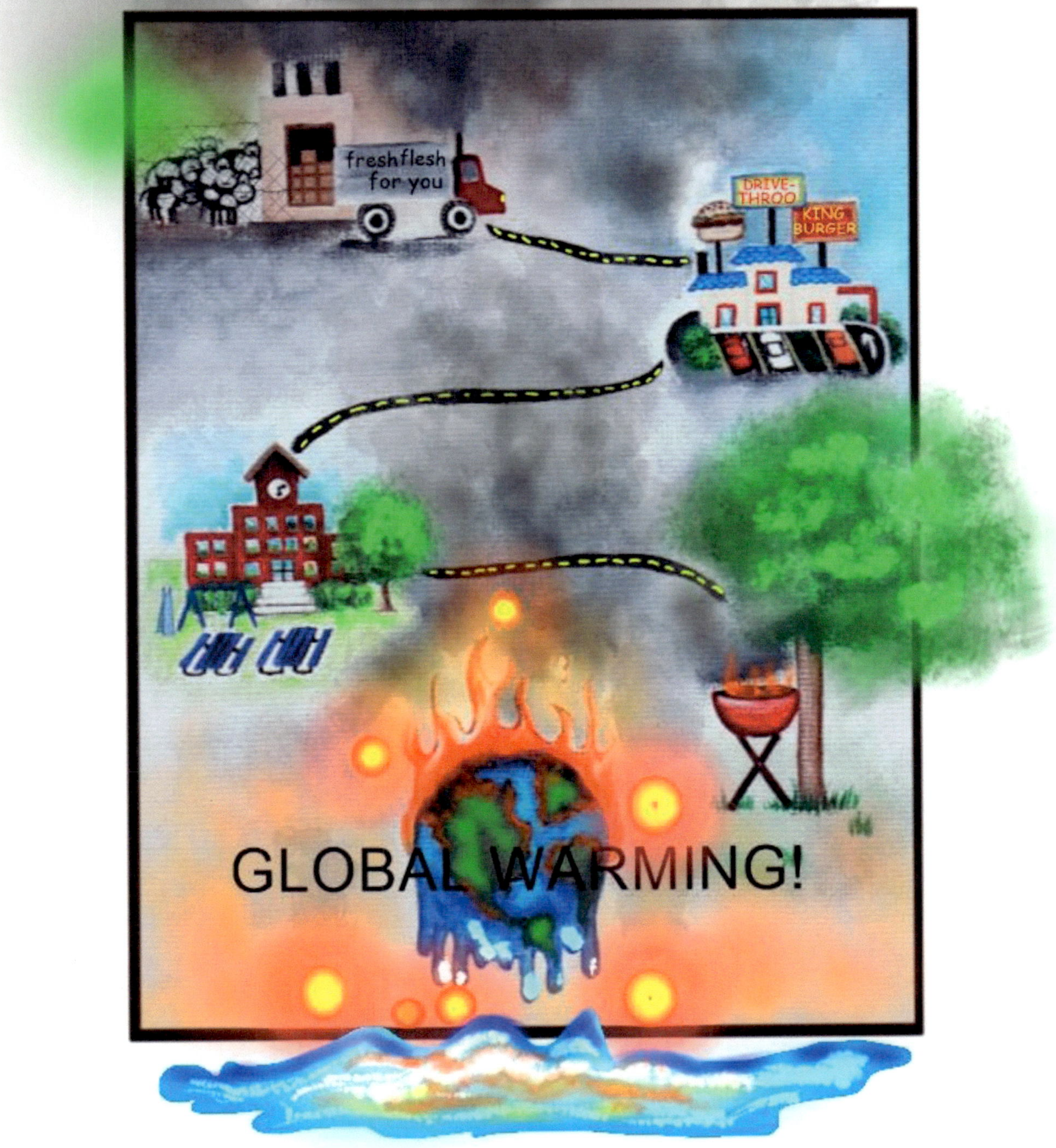

A few degrees might not sound so bad,
Coral reefs die and lose all they once had.

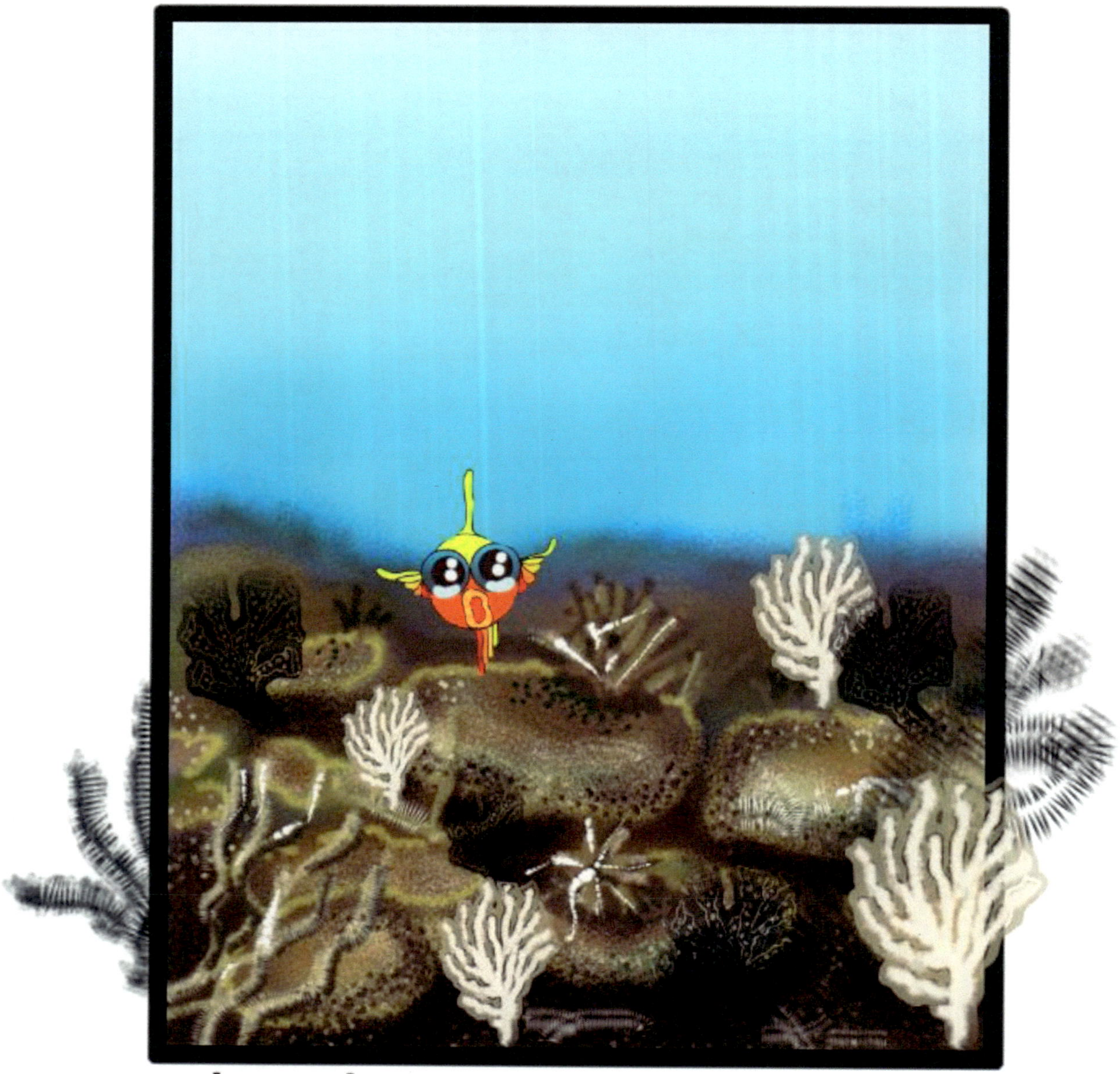

Ocean **dead zones** are nothing to scoff at,
Sea life dies from losing its habitat.

Don't I need dairy and meat to be strong?
Scientists are proving this to be wrong.

I COULD NEVER STOP EATING CHEESE

VEGETABLES ARE SO BORING

I NEED MEAT TO FEEL FULL

I CAN'T EAT MY CEREAL

ANIMALS ARE PUT ON THIS EARTH FOR FOOD

HOW WILL I GET MY PROTEIN?

ANIMALS DON'T FEEL PAIN

BUT WHAT AM I GOING TO EAT?

We can pursue a pain free tomorrow,
A **plant-based** diet will stop the sorrow.

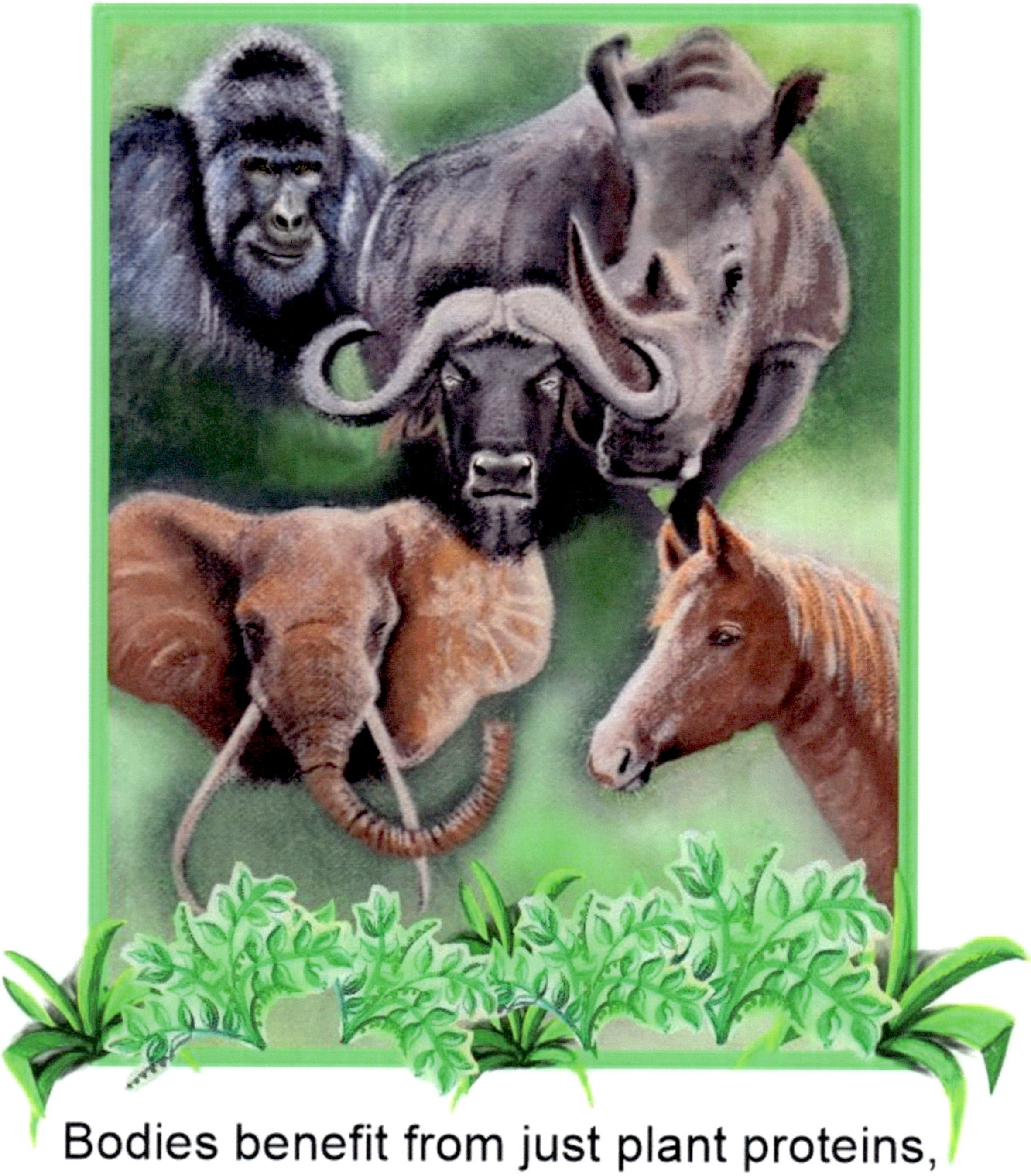

Bodies benefit from just plant proteins,
Earth's giant animals only eat greens.

Dairy and meat make arteries harden,

The **healing plants**

are grown in a garden.

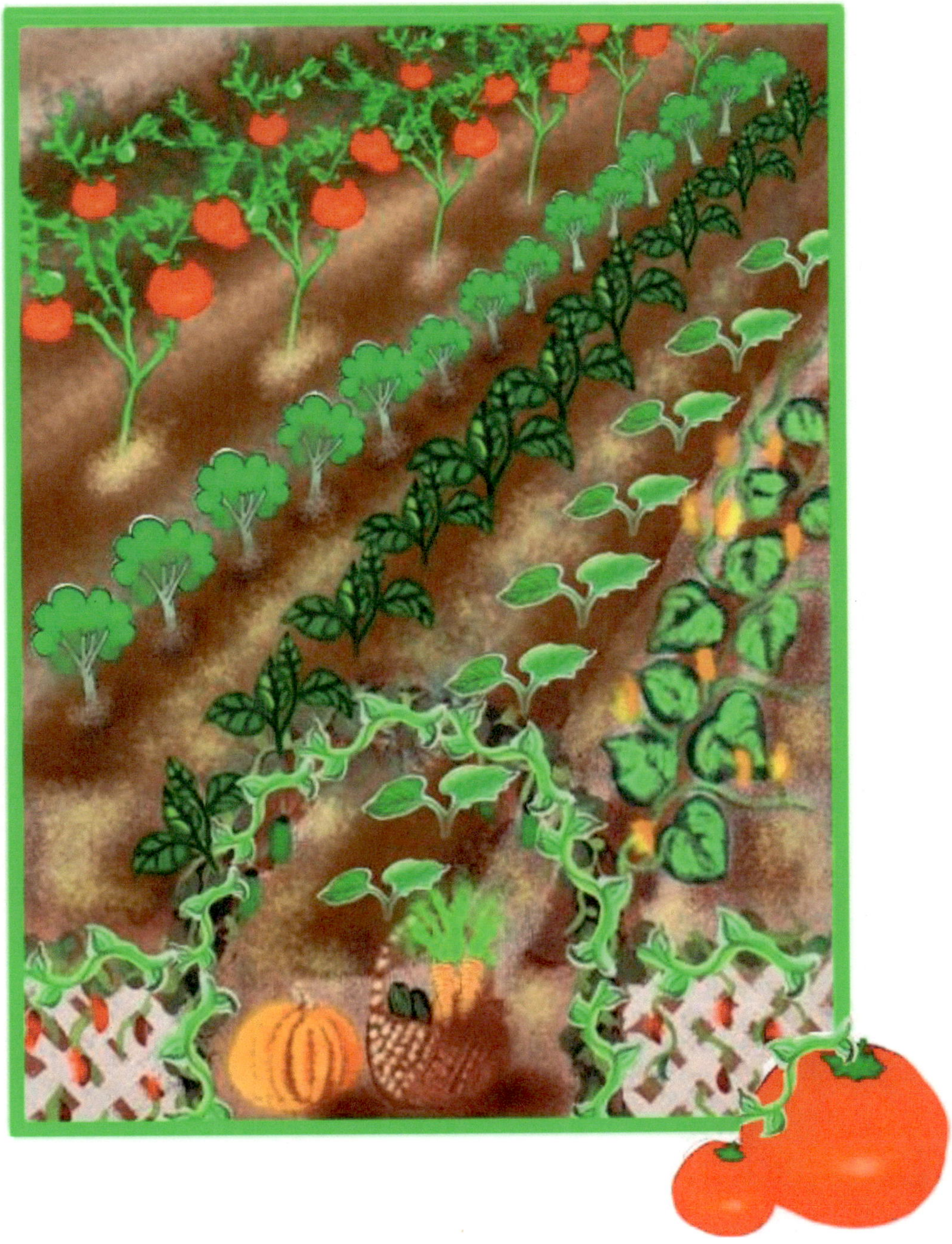

So many recipes to suit your taste,
All that require no animal waste.

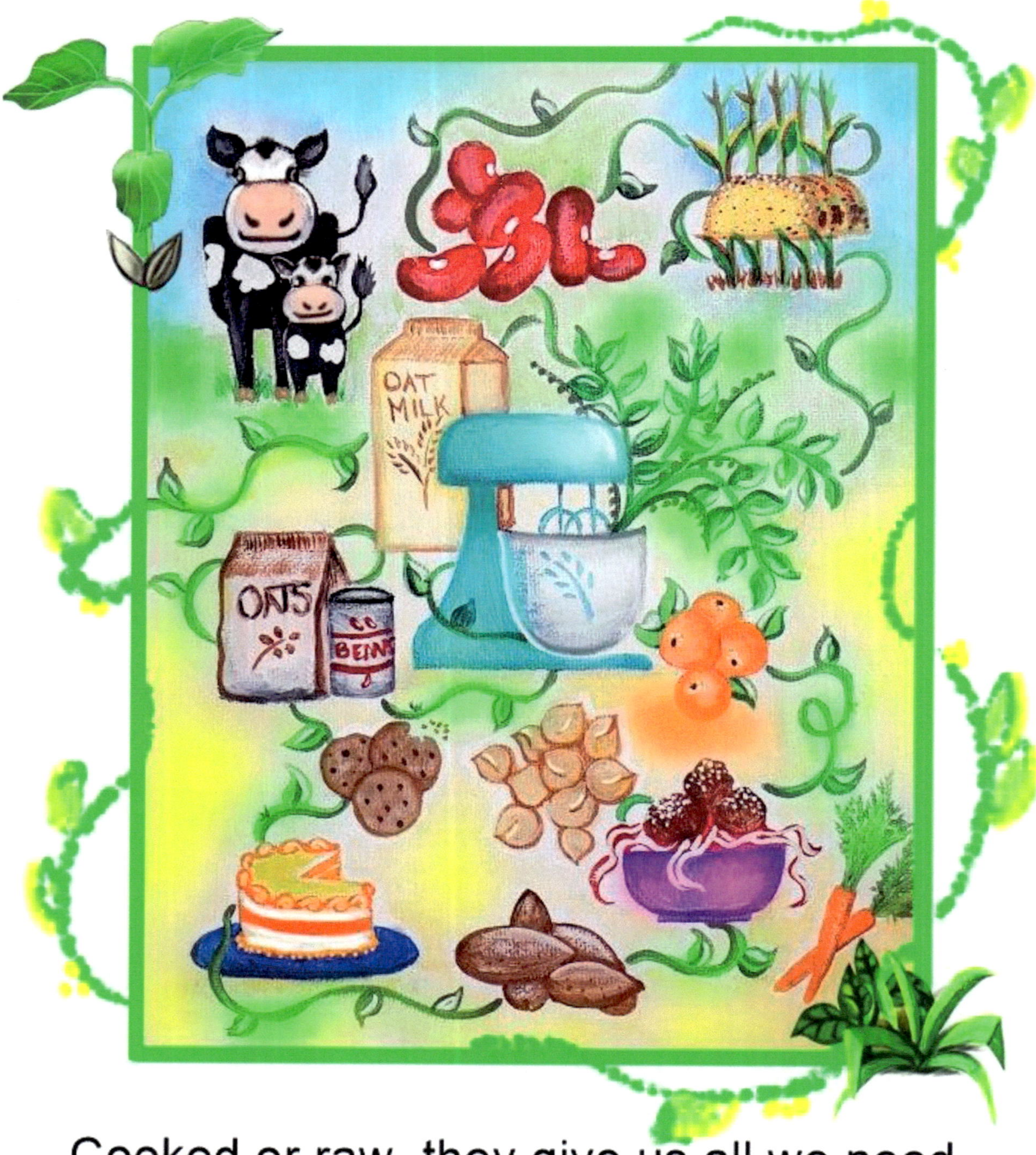

Cooked or raw, they give us all we need,
Health and prosperity grown from a seed.

So many reasons, one should not wonder,
With change, we can even cure

world hunger.

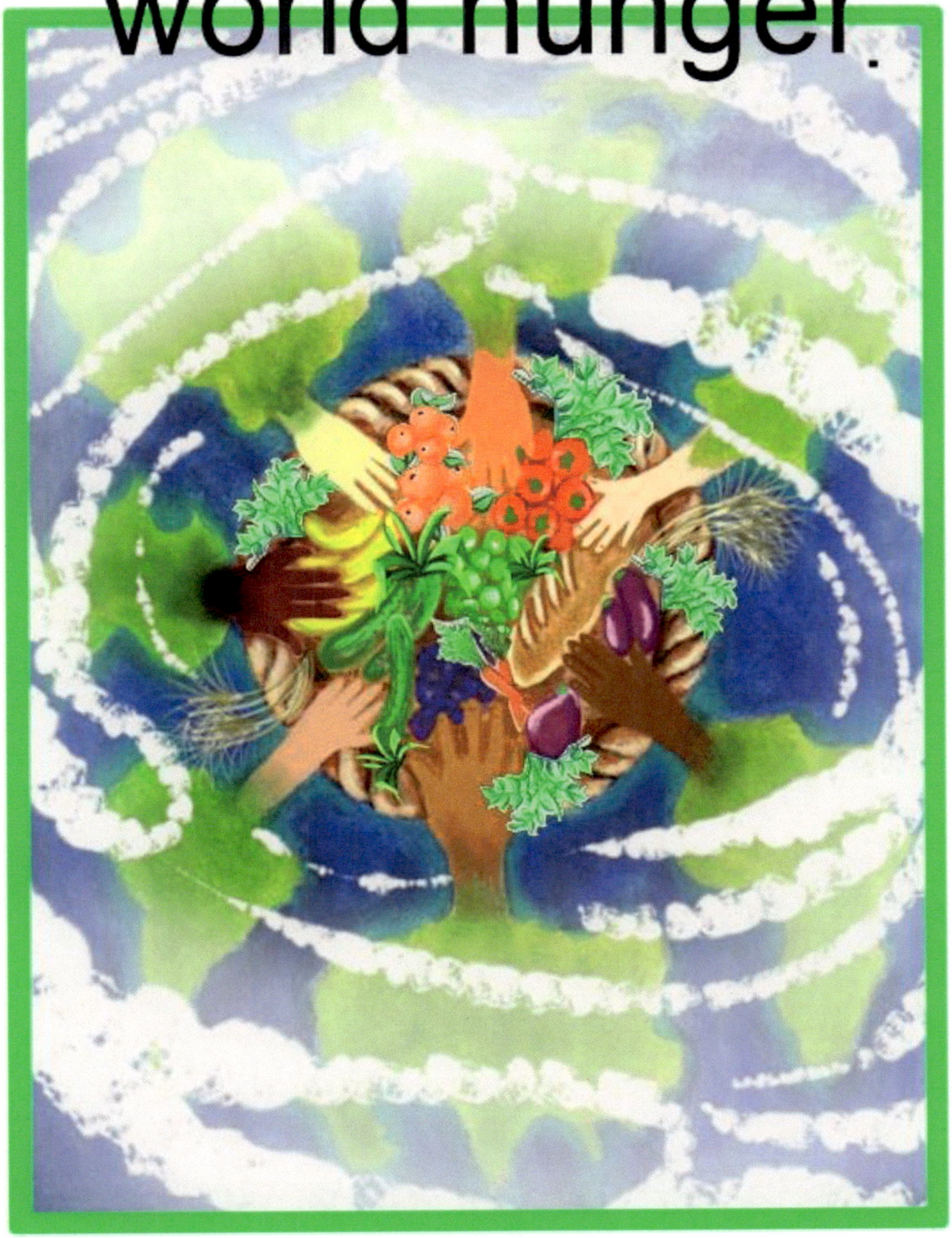

The health of our future is in each hand,
Being the solution, not the demand.

Reverse this course and make better choices,
Stop the hurt of the ones with no voices.

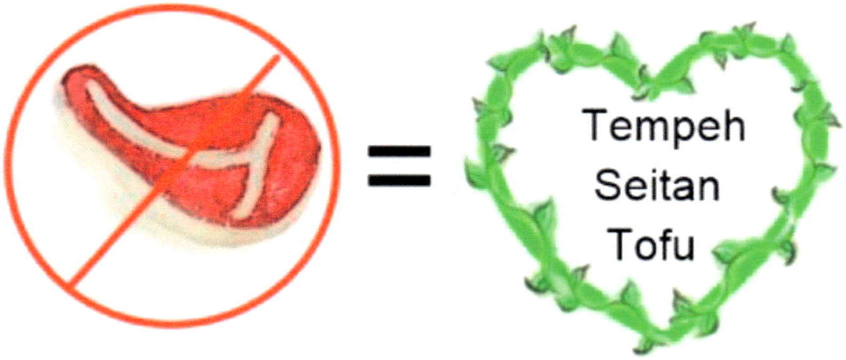

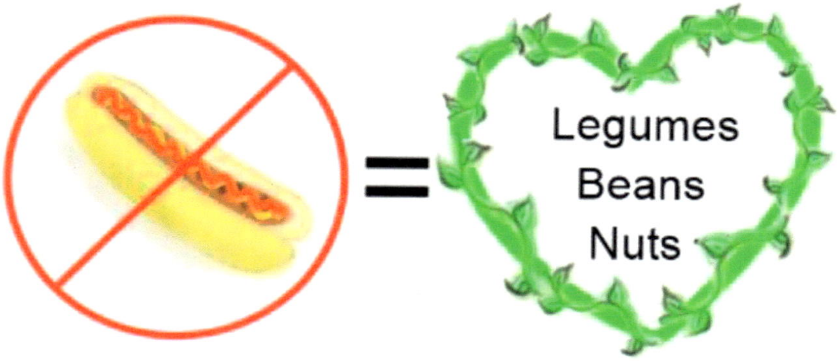

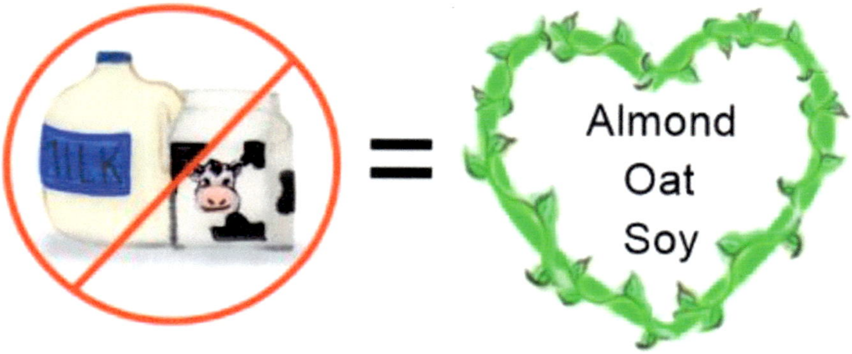

Start today and grant the cows their wish,
By choosing **no meat** for your next dish.

And when you're looking for something to munch.
please remember,

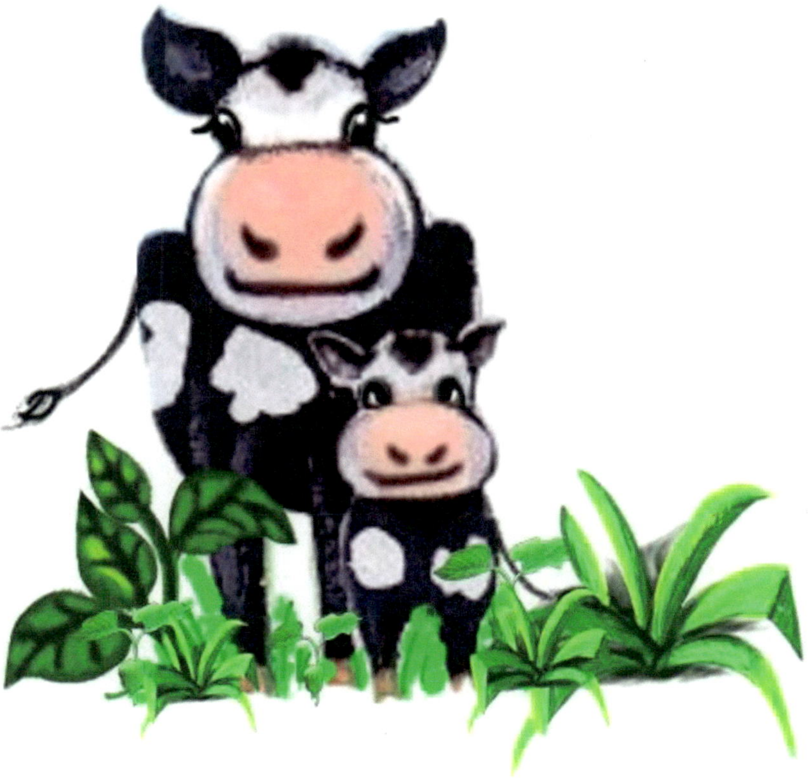

Don't have a cow, for lunch!

The End.

Beginning!

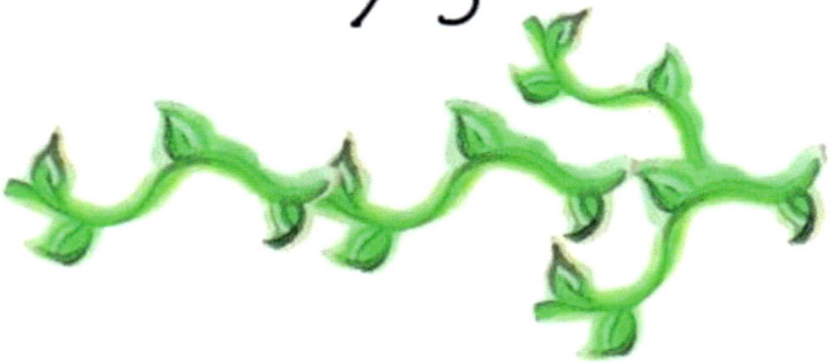

definitions

greenhouse effect the trapping of the sun's warmth in the atmosphere.

species extinction the death of the very last individual.

global warming the increase of the temperature of the earth's atmoshphere generally attributed to the greenhouse effect caused by increased levels of methane and other pollutants.

ocean dead zone areas in the ocean that fail to support the marine life living there.

ag gag bill legislation that prohibits covert documentation or investigation of conditions in the factory farming industry.

deforestation the action of clearing a wide area of trees.

prosperity the state of being wealthy, or having a rich and full life.

factory farming a system of rearing livestock using intensive methods, by which poultry, pigs, or cattle are confined indoors under strictly controlled conditions.

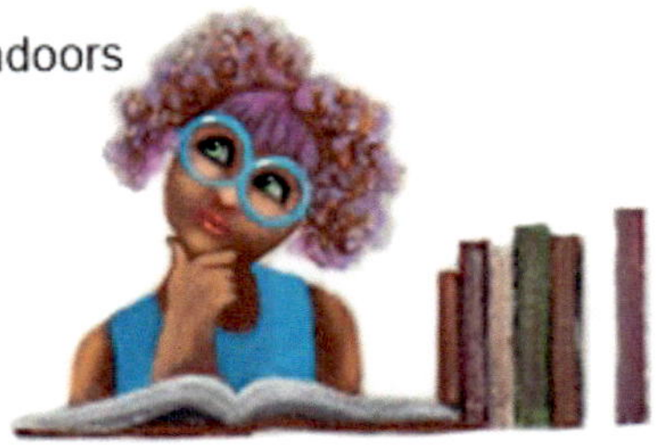

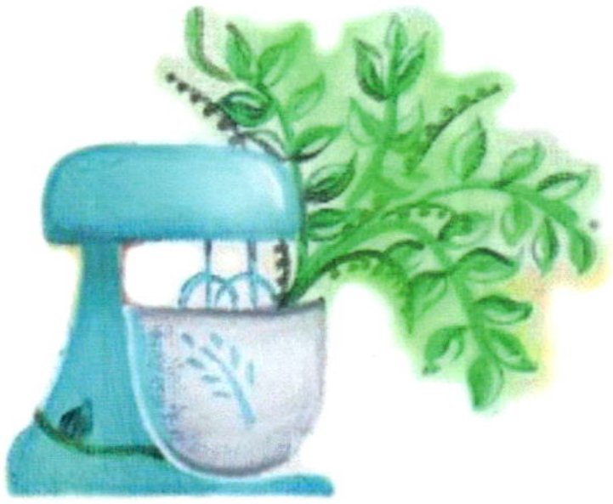

Powdered Doughed Nuts **Donuts without the refined sugar and oil!**

These dough nuts can be so many different flavors. Try adding different plant-based protein powders or nut butters! You just have to be able to roll them!

1 cup raw almonds
1 cup raw walnuts
12 pitted dates
1/3 cup pb fit
1 Tablespoon vanilla extract
5 Tablespoons water (maybe more for wetness)
1/2 teaspoon salt
1 cup oats

powdered topping:
PB Fit Peanut Butter Powder
1/4 cup granulated Monkfruit
pinch of salt

Place almonds and walnuts in a food processor and pulse to a small crumble.
Add dates, pulse again.
A vanilla, water, and salt and pulse again.
Add oats 1 cup at a time to desired consistency.
Put mixture in a bowl and mix thouroughly until dough becomes dry enough to roll.
Roll dough into a log and cut into bite size pieces. This will be your dough ball.
Once rolled into little balls, roll each ball in the PB Fit, Monkfruit, and salt.
Place in the refridgerator and try not to eat them all today!

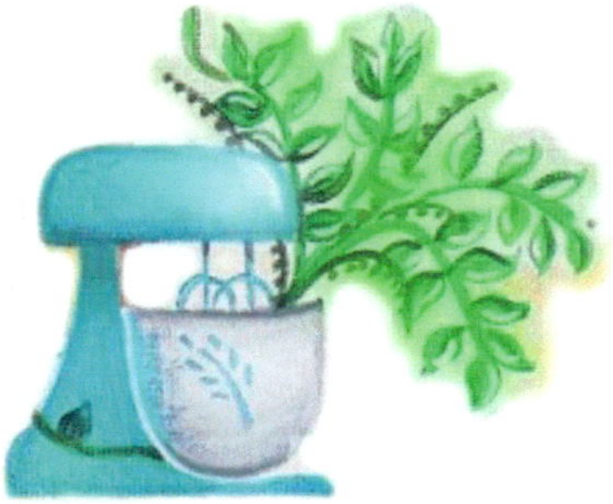

Cranberry-Chickpea "Chik'n Salad"

A favorite recipe that is super quick and easy for beginner vegans. It's gluten-free!

1 can of chickpeas (rinsed and drained)
2 ribs of celery (roughly chopped)
1/2 cup of walnuts (roughly chopped)

Blitz those ingredients together in a food processor. About 10-15 times stopping halfway to scrape down any creeping up the sideof the food processor.

Dump into a mixing bowl and add:

2 tsp dijon mustard
1 tsp yellow mustard
1/8 tsp salt
1/8 tsp pepper
1/2 cup of vegan mayo
1/2 cup of dried cranberries

Mix well until incorporated and keep refrigerated until use.

Recipe courtesy POVegan Chef (Justin Pittman)
youtube.com/POVeganChef

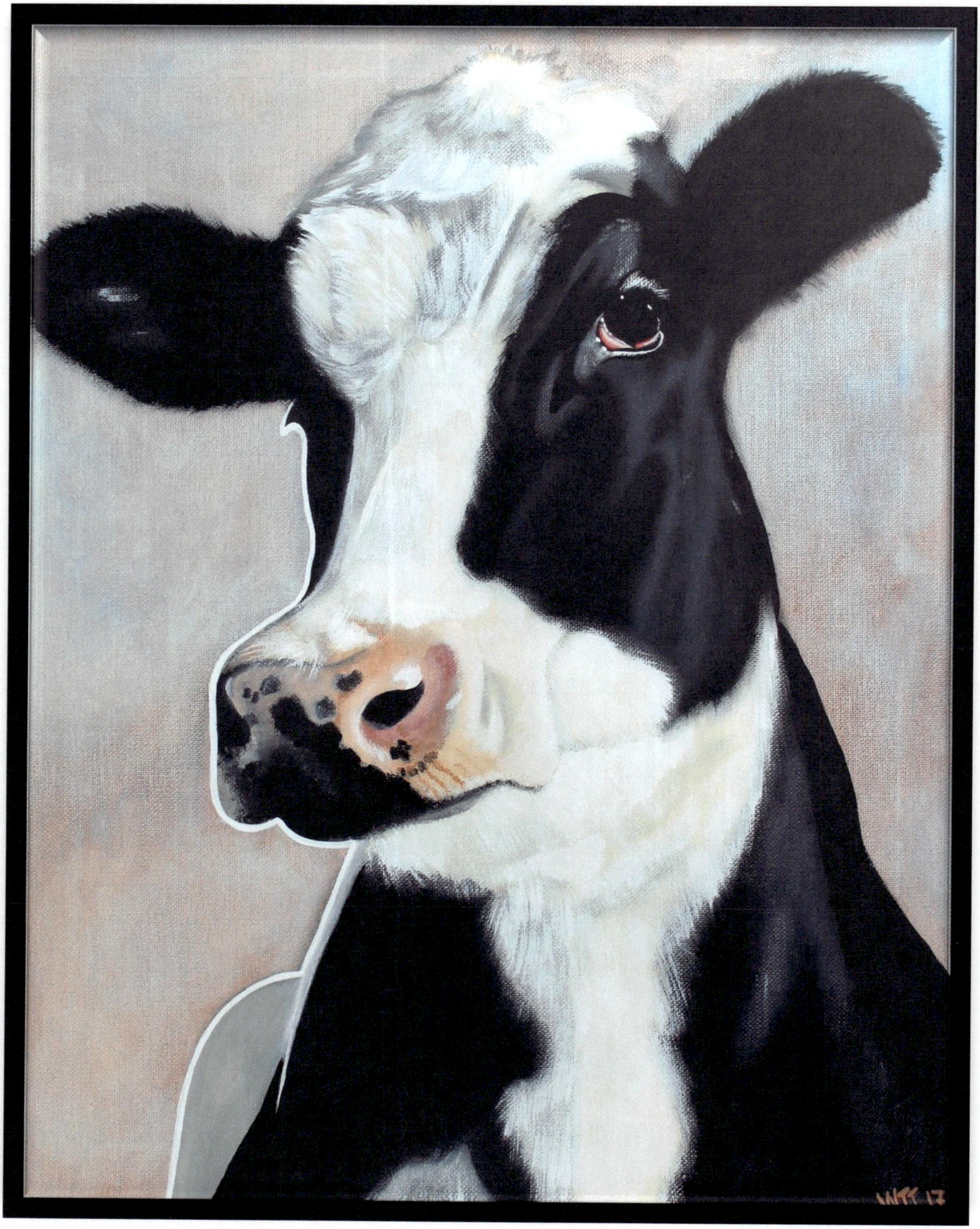

Made in the USA
Las Vegas, NV
07 November 2026

57672514R00017